Rheumatoid Arthritis

A Guide to the Natural Approach Against Rheumatoid Arthritis

Table of Contents

Introduction

What is Rheumatoid Arthritis? To be able to deal with any disease or condition, the most important thing is education. You strive to learn more about your condition so that you will understand why it's happening to you. You come face-to-face with the problem, because you want to be more capable of going against it.

This book, Rheumatoid Arthritis: A Guide to the Natural Approach against Rheumatoid Arthritis will help you deal with your condition in the healthiest and most natural way possible. It will tackle the disease, leaving nothing unturned, and then it will take the safest and most favorable route to liberation from its debilitating symptoms.

Who said you should be a slave to Rheumatoid Arthritis? Find out just how you can combat it through this book.

What Is Rheumatoid Arthritis?

A joint is the junction of two bones and its function is for movement. Arthritis is simply the inflammation of the joints.

Rheumatoid Arthritis (RA) is a chronic autoimmune disease that affects the joints. When the joints are affected, there is observed inflammation not just around the concerned area, but it has the potential to spread to the adjacent organs. When this happens, the diseased becomes a systemic illness.

What is an autoimmune disease?

These are conditions during which the body becomes under attack by its own immune system that is supposed to protect it. The immune system is the body's first line of defense. As soon as there is a foreign body, they act like soldiers, attacking the enemy in an effort to provide needed protection. When a person is said to suffer from an autoimmune disease, the patient is dealing with immune cells or antibodies that are attacking their bodies.

Ideally, the tissues within the joints secrete fluid that offers lubrication to the joints. But when a person is suffering from Rheumatoid Arthritis, the same tissues produce inflammatory material that causes loosening of the joint ligaments, as well as joint deformity. As this condition progresses, the inflammation will make matters worse, causing the erosion of bone and cartilage.

It is a chronic illness, so it can be suffered by a person for a long period of time; and they usually progress undetected, without any symptoms. Once it develops, it progresses aggressively to bring destruction to the involved structures, until it causes an obvious disability.

In the United States, about 1.3 million people suffer from Rheumatoid Arthritis and it is mostly observed in women. And the symptoms of the disease can come and go:

- Active → RA is said to be active when the tissues are inflamed

- Remission → RA is in a state of remission when the disease is inactive and the inflammation has subsided. A case of Rheumatoid Arthritis can be in remission during the course of treatment. This can extend for weeks to years, during which all symptoms disappear.

- Relapse → When the disease becomes active after a length of inactivity, you are dealing with a relapse. In this case, all the symptoms will be observed and could even flare-up.

One's experience with Rheumatoid Arthritis is different from another. The disease can go anywhere, and so subject the patient to varying experiences.

Causes and Risk Factors of Rheumatoid Arthritis

Why does one develop Rheumatoid Arthritis? Why do some people seem to fall easy victim to the condition, while some remain untouched and unaffected? A good understanding of the causes and risk factors will give light to these queries:

Causes

There is no exact trigger to bring about the development of Rheumatoid Arthritis. Regardless of what the body is dealing with, the person's immune defense become highly compromised, so that inflammation develops.

Lymphocytes are immune cells that serve as the body's first line of defense. Once activated, it releases chemical messengers such as cytokines, into the area. Basically, RA is a faulty immune response. The body assumes that there is danger, so it gives off an immune response.

Risk Factors

Anyone can become a victim of this dreaded disease. It has no age predilection, although it is most common in the elderly. Unfortunately, there are some people who can find themselves at a greater risk of developing Rheumatoid Arthritis.

The following are the known risk factors of the disease:

- Age. It can affect people, regardless of age. As a matter of fact, it can affect young individuals (juvenile idiopathic arthritis); but it is most common on individuals between the ages of 40 to 60 years old.

- Gender. It affects women, three times more than it does men.

- Genetic predisposition. It is not uncommon to find sufferers belonging to one family. This suggests that the condition had a genetic predilection and so may be passed on from parent to offspring. There are specific genes that expose the individual at a higher risk of developing RA.

- Environmental trigger. Certain exposure to environmental elements can increase one's chance of developing Rheumatoid Arthritis. Silica inhalation and excessive smoking can be misguiding the person's immune system, so that inflammation is formed.

- Microbes in the gut (bowel). Within the gut, there resides a specific type of bacteria that around found adhered to the lining of the bowels. While there is no specific microbe in question, genetically predisposed individuals find themselves victims of RA.

- Obesity. Individuals who are overweight or obese are found at a greater risk of developing rheumatoid arthritis.

Chapter 1: The Pain and Agony of Patients with Rheumatoid Arthritis

Whether you are the sufferer or you know someone who is dealing with this condition, your motivation for getting this book will depend on your direct or indirect experience with the disease. Rheumatoid arthritis is not easy to deal with—and this chapter will discuss this aspect, closely.

Signs and Symptoms

The most significant issue that patients deal with Rheumatoid Arthritis relates to the pain and discomfort involved with incurring the disease. How does Rheumatoid Arthritis affect your life? What symptoms are you struggling with? The following are the known signs and symptoms:

- Joint and muscle stiffness. After a long period of inactivity, the muscles and joints usually feel stiff. Also referred to as post-sedentary stiffness, it is common in the morning, upon waking up. This is most common with all sufferers.

- Swelling, tenderness, pain and redness of joints. Observed, most especially, during disease flares, the joints exhibit swelling, tenderness, pain and redness because the synovium (lining of the joint tissues) are exceedingly inflamed. There is noted increased production of synovial fluid and thickening of the synovium, referred to as synovitis.

- Polyarthritis. Due to its symmetrical occurrence in the body, it is often referred to as symmetric polyarthritis. It is highly differentiated from other types of arthritis, such as Osteoarthritis, that may occur on one side of the body.

- Immobility and loss of joint function. Due to muscle and joint stiffness, the small joints of the hands and feet present some difficulty of movement. Even small range of movements such as twisting, bending and turning of joints will be impossible. At the same time, walking can become painful and quite labored.

- Loss of muscle function. When the inflammation is prolonged, this causes damage to the adjacent tissues, such as the bone and cartilage. Damage to bone and cartilage will lead to muscle weakness, a decrease in the range of motion, and even the loss of function. This will greatly affect the person's daily existence.

- Hoarseness of voice. The cricoarytenoid joint is in charge of the tightening of the vocal cords, for the production of various sounds. When the inflammation is found in the area of the vocal cords, there is an observed alteration to voice tone.

- Fever, fatigue and weight loss. Due to the chronic inflammation, patients with RA are found to be fatigued, losing appetite and eventually, losing weight, over the course of the development of the disease. Inflammation can cause the patient to develop a fever, thus a rise in temperature may be expected.

Patients can deal with a few or all of these symptoms. But note that when they occur, they are found to affect the both side of the body, in perfect symmetry. If you are dealing with these symptoms, the next thing you need to do is to rule out other conditions.

Differentiating Rheumatoid Arthritis from Other Diseases

The symptoms of Rheumatoid Arthritis are easily confused as some other condition. To properly address your problem, it is important that you identify what disease you are really dealing with.

The following are some of the conditions that appear like Rheumatoid Arthritis:

1. Gout and Pseudogout. Gout involves asymmetric oligoarticular and monoarticular arthritis with inflammation that can span for about 3-10 days. In the case of Pseudogout, the symptoms to be dealt with appear like gout, rheumatoid arthritis, or osteoarthritis, but involve CPPD crystal deposition.

2. Fibromylagia. There is stiffness when at rest, as well as the presence of symmetrical arthtralgias; however, this condition does not present with pain or synovitis.

3. Lupus. SLE can present with symptoms that involve disability that mimics that of RA, however, the problem is not with the joints but the ligament and tendon.

4. Osteoarthritis. It is a non-inflammatory disease that involves the thinning of the joint cartilage. Unlike the characteristic symmetry that may be observed with cases of RA, symptoms of Osteoarthritis may affect just one side of the body (one knee or one elbow).

5. Post-Viral Arthritis. Acute and chronic viral infections present with polyarthritis that looks very much like RA.

6. Sarcoidosis. A patient with this condition may or may not test positive in the RF Test and will present with synovitis, but a tissue biopsy can further differentiate it from RA.

7. Seronegative Spondyloarthritis. Especially when there is no rash, psoriatic arthritis can be confused with RA. The same is true with the other seronegative spondyloarthropathies, but the symptoms are often asymmetrical.

8. Vasculitis. The symptoms of giant cell carcinoma and polymyalgia rheumatica include symmetrical polyarthritis.

Complications of Rheumatoid Arthritis

Rheumatoid Arthritis typically starts in the joints. Inflammation develops within the joints, but a negative progression of the disease can also affect different organs, like the eyes or the lungs.

Severe cases of RA can become a systemic problem. This leads to:

1. Sjogren's syndrome. This involved inflammation of the optic glands and dryness of the mouth.

2. Corneal abrasion. Due to excessive dryness of the eyes, it can lead to corneal damage.

3. Scleritis. This is the inflammation of the sclerae (white of the eye) and can be very critical to overall eye health.

4. Pleuritis. When the inflammation in the joints spread to the lining of the lungs, one develops pleuritis that is characterized by severe chest pain. The patient will experience shortness of breath, coughing, and difficulty of breathing.

5. Rheumatoid nodules. As a result of the inflammation in the lining of the lungs, the tissues can become scarred and inflamed, so that nodules develop within the

surface. These nodules can also develop on the elbows and fingers, and are tender to pressure.

6. Pericarditis. When the inflammation spreads, it can cause inflammation of the tissues surrounding the heart. This is characterized by severe pain in the chest that is mostly felt when the person is leaning forward or lying down. Progression of this condition may also lead to heart attack.

7. Anemia. Prolonged cases of RA can lead to a rapid decrease in the number of both red blood cells and white blood cells.

8. Fety's syndrome. Due to the rapid decrease of white blood cells, the patient can develop a large spleen and become exceedingly prone to infection.

9. Lymphoma. Cases of lymphoma are found quite common in patient suffering from Rheumatoid Arthritis.

10. Carpal tunnel syndrome. This is a condition that results from the nerves becoming pinched due to pressure from the inflammatory elements.

11. Vasculitis. When the patient suffers RA for long time, the blood vessels can also become inflamed. When this happens, vascular supply is compromised and may lead to necrosis or tissue death. It usually appears as black areas around the leg or nail beds.

Chapter 2: Diagnosis and Treatment of Rheumatoid Arthritis

While signs and symptoms usually signify the presence of a condition, it is not definitive. There is so much about Rheumatoid Arthritis than meets the eye; and this section of the book will attempt to bring you even closer.

Diagnosis of Rheumatoid Arthritis

How does one know if for certain that the problem they are dealing with is, indeed, Rheumatoid Arthritis?

1. RA Test or RF Test. There is an antibody called the "rheumatoid factor" that is present in the blood of 80% of those who suffer from Rheumatoid Arthritis. This antibody is easy detected through a blood test. The RA Test or RG Test will detect the presence of rheumatoid factor in the blood. It is possible to have Rheumatoid Arthritis, while testing negative for the rheumatoid factor. A patient testing positive to this test has "seropositive rheumatoid arthritis" and those who test negative to it has "serogenative rheumatoid arthritis"

2. Citrulline Antibody Test. There is another antibody called the "citrulline antibody" that is present in 50% of those who suffer from Rheumatoid Arthritis. It is also called the anti-citrulline antibody, anti-CCP antibody, or anticyclic citrullinated peptide antibody, and when the patient does not present with the common symptoms of RA, this is the definitive test. It may also be used for seronegative rheumatoid arthritis patients.

3. Sedimentation Rate. This is a special blood test that can be used to measure the rate of inflammation in the joints. After extracting blood from the patient, the rate of sedimentation or the speed at which the RBC drops to the bottom of the tube is recorded. Sed Rate is high in active cases of RA and lowest during remission.

4. C - reactive protein Test. Apart from its use for RA, this test is also useful in the detection of anemia. Chronic inflammation due to Rheumatoid Arthritis is almost always synonymous to occurrences anemia.

5. ANA Test. The antinuclear antibody test detects the presence of the ANA in the body to confirm Rheumatoid Arthritis.

6. Radiographic Test. X-ray tests of the affected areas will signify the presence of any changes in the joints or any nodules formed, as a result of the inflammation. The disease brings various changes that are detectable by radiofrequency, such as erosion of bone.

7. MRI. Magnetic Resonance Imaging may be used to scan bone. Radioactive substance, even at a small amount, can detect the inflammation of the joints.

8. Arthrocentesis. Using a needle and a syringe, some fluid is drained from the inflamed joint, so that it may be assessed in a laboratory. A test such as this will help differentiate RA from gout or infection.

When a patient comes in, complaining about RA, the physician or rheumatologist (specialist) will interview the patient to uncover the family and medical history. The symptoms will be discussed, and depending whatever is already obvious, either of the tests mentioned above will be performed.

To eliminate confusion with other conditions, a differentiation will be performed to rule out gout or other forms of arthritis.

Stages of Rheumatoid Arthritis

To say that RA is a complicated disease is an understatement, but the best way to classify the disease is to grade it according to how it appears in a radiographic test. The classifications will more or less, describe the progression of the disease:

Stage I
- Minimal bone thinning with no significant damage

Stage II
- Notable bone thinning on the proximity of the joint but there is no significant damage
- There may be some damage to cartilage
- There may difficulty in movement but there are no defects on the joint
- Atrophy of the adjacent muscle due to severing inflammation
- Deformities on the adjacent soft tissues

Stage III
- Evident bone thinning and notable damage on the bone and cartilage
- Deformity of the joint with some reversible immobility and stiffening
- Severe atrophy of muscles
- Abnormalities on the adjacent soft tissues

Stage IV
- Osteoporosis evident around the joint and notable damage on the bone and cartilage
- Deformity of the joint with ankylosis (permanent immobility and fixation)
- Severe atrophy of muscles
- Abnormalities on the adjacent soft tissues

Traditional Treatments and Medications

There is no definite cure for Rheumatoid Arthritis. Most of the treatment modalities are designed to help the patient survive the symptoms. It reduces pain and inflammation, so that damage to the structures is prevented, and function and movement may be restored.

Traditional Treatments

Treatment, therefore, will be matched to the specific need that demands it.

1. Arthrocentesis. While this is traditionally used as a diagnostic test, this may also be used as a treatment. Liberating some of the inflammatory material in the joints can bring some relief, so that conditions may be improved.

2. Arthroscopy. When there is an obvious deformity in the joints, it may be resolved by surgery. Whether some partial or complete repair is required, arthroscopy allows the surgeon to insert and instrument to manipulate the damaged joints.

3. Joint replacement. When the joints are severely damaged to utter destruction, an artificial replacement may be required. This is common to knee joints and hip joints.

Medications

First Line Drugs
These include aspirin and cortisone. Cortisone is occasionally combined with arthrocentesis for pain relief. Steroids can deal with the pain and the swelling caused by inflammation. It can also deal with other symptoms. Also in this category are your NSAIDs because they can deal with symptoms of inflammation. They basically deal with pain and inflammation, so that patients may be relieved from the excruciating symptoms of the disease.

Second Line Drugs

They are slow-acting drugs and are also known as DMARDs (Disease Modifying Antirheumatic Drugs). These include methotrexate and hydroxychlorine and as second line of defense their action helps in prevention and initiation of remission.

Dealing with the Complications

When the problem is not exactly in the joints, but is supposed to deal with a complication that has resulted from prolonged RA, the following medications will be required:

- Eye drops for drying of the eyes due to Sjogren's syndrome.

- Cortisone injections for rheumatoid nodules, bursitis, and tendinitis.

- Oral cortisone for lung inflammation

Unfortunately, there is still no absolute cure for Rheumatoid Arthritis. There is only a means of managing the symptoms, so that one can continue with their lives, with as much comfort as possible.
The traditional treatments and medications mentioned in this chapter are the not the only options you have. As a matter of fact, they are not the best options you have.

Chapter 3: All-Natural Treatment of Rheumatoid Arthritis

The symptoms of Rheumatoid Arthritis vary from one person to another. The necessity of the treatment is often dictated by the severity of the present symptoms. Your experience increases the need for treatment, and before anything is obtained, a physician or rheumatologist will classify the symptoms accordingly:

Class I: Still able to perform, normal day-to-day life activities, with much ease and comfort

Class II: Still able to perform normal day-to-day life activities, but only those that falls under personal care and work. Sports and more engaging household chores will be more difficult.

Class III: Still able to perform normal day-to-day life activities, but only those that falls under personal care. Work and other activities will be more difficult.

Class IV: No longer able to perform normal day-to-day life activities, even personal care.

Benefits of Going Natural

When a person is ill, the automatic response is to pop a pill. Everyone is most accustomed to turning to medications without realizing that there are safer and more effective means of addressing their condition.

1. Reduced risk against harmful side-effects. In the next section, you will come face-to-face with the long list of side effects that you can suffer from the use of over-the-counter medications. It's almost part and parcel of the whole decision to take medications. You take it to be able to address a specific issue, but as you do so, you put yourself at risk of developing other problems. But while natural remedies are not without side effects, they are easier to handle. A close attention to dosing will be a good safety net against the ill effects of some natural remedies.

2. It promotes natural body healing. Many of the natural remedies function to stimulate production and secretion of specific substances already present in the body. Sometimes, a malfunction or defect will cause a decrease in the normal production of said substances; but with proper stimulation, failures in the body's normal physiological processes will be corrected, and the body deals with its own triggers—as designed by nature.

3. It is more affordable. Over-the-counter medications have gone through series of research and laboratory testing and manufacturers and distributors spend so much money for these substances. The economics involved in the sale of various medications have been an accepted fact. Patients all over the world endure heightened fees of medicines because they feel they have no other choice. Fortunately, natural remedies give patients a more cost-effective option to deal with their symptoms. Some of the substances are cooking

recipes you have lying around in the house, so it will not even incur extra expense for you.

4. It is most effective, especially in chronic conditions. The problem with Rheumatoid Arthritis is that it can be a lifelong problem. Since there is no definite cure, most cases become a chronic condition. In this case, natural remedies become a better address for symptoms of RA because they are proven safer.

5. It is readily available. Compared to over-the-counter medications that need to be bought; and some exclusively acquired from specific companies, natural remedies are market finds. Some are available in the grocery and may be incorporated into daily routines and rituals. Some herbs and spices can be combined with food and beverage; and some require manipulation to form various oral and topical concoctions.

6. They are clean. The raw materials are things you see in your kitchen. These are substances you use to cook your food or to make your tea. You probably have some of it from time-to-time without realizing its good effects for your health. They are not manufactured in the laboratory. They are not synthetic. They are pure and natural; therefore, they are clean.

7. They are milder. Over-the-counter medications make use of substances that are potent and so have the potential to bring some harm to the body. Natural ingredients may not be as strong, but at least you can rest assured that it is not going to bring you direct harm. Of course, some caution is placed on the strict dosing instructions, but other than that, you can trust for natural ingredients to be kinder, milder, and more caring.

8. They address more than one condition. You may think you are merely addressing Rheumatoid Arthritis, but most natural ingredients can provide resolution to a myriad of things. This means that you are going to successful hit not just two birds with one stone, but possibly dozens. In the ancient times, there was no over-the-counter medication manufactured in laboratories. People relied on natural substances and they were meant to address not just one but two or more conditions.

The most significant thing you have to realize is that there is no specific cure for Rheumatoid Arthritis. To live through the symptoms, you have to address it in a long-term point of view. Popping pills may resolve a temporary symptom, but are you going to pop the pill for the rest of your life? Dealing with RA the natural way is going to be most ideal. Altering your lifestyle, so that it is fits with your condition, is the best way to go.

The Risk of Traditional Medications and Treatment Modalities

If you really want to understand how important it is to take a natural approach when tackling Rheumatoid Arthritis.
You may want to look into the various side effects of traditional treatments and medications:

- Abdominal pain
- Bone marrow damage
- Cataracts
- Diarrhea
- Easy bruising
- Facial puffiness
- Fever and chills
- Gastrointestinal bleeding
- Hair loss
- Increased risk of infection

- Kidney damage
- Metallic taste in the mouth
- Mouth sores
- Muscle wasting
- Reduced liver function and cirrhosis
- Skins rashes and allergies
- Upset stomach
- Ulcers
- Vision problems
- Weight gain

Now that you have come face-to-face with the awful truth, what do you plan to do? The next chapters go into detail with the natural remedies for Rheumatoid Arthritis.

Who said you have to be a slave to over-the-counter medications, all your life? Living with RA doesn't have to be so unbearable. Find out just how to take better control of your condition, in the next chapters.

Chapter 4: Natural Treatments for Rheumatoid Arthritis

Medications are everyone's first though when it comes to illnesses, but with the increasing awareness about the effects of various substances in the body, more people are making the "natural choice".

In the case of Rheumatoid Arthritis, you choose to go the natural route because natural treatments are gentler and safer. They are just as effective if not more effective as medicines.

Herbs and Spices against Rheumatoid Arthritis

Herbs and Spices are considered homeopathic treatments. They are more readily available compared to medicines; and they are more affordable. Why do you have to go through painful surgeries when you can manage your condition with natural ingredients?

1. Black Pepper. A readily available and popular table spice, but it is not very known that it has healing properties against inflammation and pain. It contains capsaicin, a component common to anti-inflammatory creams and lotions, so it is very effective for pain relief in Rheumatoid Arthritis.

2. Boswellia Serrata. This plant releases a sap or resin, called frankincense, which is a popular anti-inflammatory agent that has the ability to suppress the autoimmune response related to the onset of RA. But to maximize the effects of this plant, it is best to combine it with organic grade turmeric. It is also believed to help prevent the loss of cartilage.

3. Cat's Claw. Uncaria tomentosa is an effective anti-inflammatory agent that can suppress the action of the tumor necrosis factor (TNF). Taken in regulation, in

can be very beneficial to the immune system and it will be very reliable in swelling and joint pain.

4. Cinnamon. More than the amazing aroma and distinctive taste, a cinnamon bark has anti-inflammatory properties that can help with pain relief. Just as long as you take this in moderation, it can be very good for various cases of Rheumatoid Arthritis.

5. Coriander. A staple ingredient for various Thai and Mexican dishes that has anti-inflammatory properties.

6. Green Tea. A well known anti-inflammatory agent, it contains polyphenols and powerful antioxidants that have the ability to suppress the malfunctioning of the immune system which causes Rheumatoid Arthritis. Commonly enjoyed as a hot cuppa, green tea definitely goes a long way in terms of just being a beverage.

7. Turmeric. This is a yellow "ginger-like" spice that is mostly used for curry dishes. Unknown to many, it can be very effective for the relief of various symptoms of Rheumatoid Arthritis. Especially when taken in its organic oil or pill form, you take advantage of the CO_2 extraction, where turmeric is in its cleanest and purest form. There are no additives, fillers, or artificial ingredients.

8. Willow Bark. The bark of a willow tree has anti-inflammatory properties. It is similar to aspirin, and is able to bring pain relief, but some caution is placed on the dosing of willow bark because it contains salicin. The substance, salicin, is capable of shutting down kidney function when taken in large doses. As a matter of fact, it is known that the musician Beethhoven died of salicin overdose.

Note well that dosage is very critical when perusing any of the substances listed here. The best address, therefore, is to transform your diet so that you enjoy the following substance in moderation (as used and applied to your meals).

The next chapters will go into further detail about food and diet; as well as its role in the treatment and management of Rheumatoid Arthritis.

Home Remedies for Rheumatoid Arthritis

Risks Involved with Natural Remedies

To make an informed decision, it is important that you have a good grasp of the world of natural remedies; because while it presents with amazing benefits, they also come with some risks:

- Risk of poison due to dosing. Proper dosing for natural ingredients can be a little tricky and if patients are not careful, there is risk of poison. Some cases of overdose from certain herbs and spices can even be fatal, if you are not very careful. This means that success with the use of such substance rely on thorough research and religious following of strict instructions. It is easy to take a misstep but it is also possible to be on the safe side, just as long as you know and understand what you are doing.

- Drug interactions. If you are currently taking over-the-counter medications for other conditions, not related to Rheumatoid Arthritis, you have to look into any known drug interactions. Some herbs and spices have interactions with prescription medications, so you need to be wary about these things.

- Allergies. The body can react to certain substances, differently than others do. And you have to watch out for any allergies to substances that you may have, and so bring you harm.

- Lack of regulation. It is readily available and almost obtained everywhere so there is not much regulation in terms of quality. Unless you take time to make a thorough research on where it is best to acquire your natural ingredients from, it is very easy to fall into inferior brands, batches, or manufacturers.

In the next chapters, you will take through the more practical approaches available for the management of symptoms related to Rheumatoid Arthritis.
It calls for a massive lifestyle alteration, but it is very reliable if it is observed religiously.

Chapter 5: Rheumatoid Arthritis and Your Diet

Do you know the food that you put into your mouth, has the ability to direct the course of your bout with Rheumatoid Arthritis? They did not say "you are what you eat, for nothing". Your food choices ultimately translate to the kind of life your will live, being that you are suffering from RA.

The symptoms of Rheumatoid Arthritis can be very tough to handle. It causes debilitating pain and it has the capacity to change one's life, so it is pertinent that you find a means to cope. If caring for what you eat is going to change your whole story, altogether, then you have start minding your plate.

Foods to Avoid

Everyone loves to eat. But if your food choices are giving you a hard time, then perhaps you should look closely into your diet:

- Alcohol. While alcohol is not completely bad, studies show that people who drank more than three glasses of alcohol in a week put themselves at a greater risk of developing Rheumatoid Arthritis. C-reactive protein, a known marker of inflammation, is said to increase with high consumption of alcohol. This means that if you want to deal with the debilitating symptoms of RA, you will refrain from taking too much alcohol.

- Carbohydrates. Refined sugar and flour are the most problematic carbs for people with Rheumatoid Arthritis because it can raise blood sugar levels that will cause the overproduction of cytokines. Cytokines are inflammatory chemicals that will only worsen the symptoms of RA.

- Coffee. A cup of coffee is essential to many people's lives because they cannot function without it. Unfortunately, you might want to switch to a cup of tea, instead or perhaps, go for black coffee. Heavy coffee drinking may keep you going but it will also increase your risk of developing Rheumatoid Arthritis.

- Diet soda. Beverages such as diet soda contain a large amount of aspartame. This substance is known to trigger inflammation so patients suffering from Rheumatoid Arthritis are only putting themselves at risk.

- Fried food. Fried foods are heavy on harmful toxins, advanced glycation end products that can cause an increased oxidation in the body. When this happens, there is higher risk for inflammation.

- Gluten. This is a type of protein that is sourced from certain grains such as barley, rye, and wheat. Gluten increases the risk for the development of various autoimmune diseases, such as Rheumatoid Arthritis.

- MSG. A well-known food additive, monosodium glutamate is a chemical based substance that is known to increase the risk of developing inflammatory diseases such as Rheumatoid Arthritis. When a person offers from RA, their immune defense is down and at times, food substances such as MSG will be noted as a foreign body so that inflammation will ensue in an effort to attack it.

- Processed foods. It doesn't matter if you suffer from RA or not, processed foods are bad news because they are heavy on harmful substances that will only increase your risk of developing inflammation.

- Red meat. Red meat is rich in saturated fat and omega-6 fatty acids that will only make inflammation a bigger problem. Patients with RA observed great improvement in their condition when they cut red meat from their diet. This doesn't mean that you have to cut meat, completely, because you just have to go lean.

- Salt. While salt is not entirely bad, having it in excess is going to be detrimental for you and your Rheumatoid Arthritis. Salt can cause a spike in your blood pressure and when there is a high level of sodium in your blood, you become more prone to developing autoimmune disorders such as RA.

Foods to Enjoy

- Beans. Rich in fiber and protein, which is good for muscle health, beans can help lower the amount of C-reactive protein in the blood, which a know market for inflammation. Good sources are pinto beans, red beans, and kidney beans.

- Blackstrap molasses. Rich in vitamins and minerals, especially magnesium which is responsible for the preservation of muscle, nerve, and cartilage health. People with RA are often found with a deficiency in magnesium, so supplying your diet with enough sources of magnesium will counter the bad condition.

- Broccoli. Cruciferous vegetables such as broccoli I not only healthy, but for a patient suffering from Rheumatoid Arthritis, they can enjoy a significant decrease in the onset of inflammatory symptoms. It contains sulfurophane that specifically blocks the onset of inflammation.

  Recommended consumption is about 2 to 3 cups of vegetables per meal

- Cherries. Rich in anthocyanins, cherries like blueberries, raspberries, strawberries, and blackberries have very reliable anti-inflammatory properties. So they are very good against inflammation caused by Rheumatoid Arthritis. Cherries are also known to decrease the levels of nitric oxide in the body, a compound found to be responsible for the onset of Rheumatoid Arthritis.

Recommended consumption is about 1 ½ to 2 cups of fruits per meal

- Dairy products. Rich in vitamin D and calcium, low fat dairy can boost the function of the immune system so that it does not fail. Rheumatoid Arthritis happens to the failure of the immune system. With ample supply of low fat dairy products, you help prevent the onset of RA.

- Fish. Omega-3 fatty acids can block prostaglandins and cytokines. Not only that, it can convert these two potentially harmful substances into anti-inflammatory chemicals known as resolvins. In these forms, patients are able to receive help against joint stiffness and tenderness. The best sources of fish oil and omega-3 fatty acids are tuna, mackerel, salmon, and herring.

Recommended consumption is about 3-4 oz (twice a week).

- Garlic. A common ingredient used in the kitchen, garlic is not only a tasty vegetable, but it has anti-inflammatory properties that help in pain relief for Rheumatoid Arthritis. Its effectiveness in inflammation is due to the production of cytokines that helps suppress the onset of inflammation. Note well that garlic's prowess is best enjoyed in its raw form because once it is cooked; some of its nutritious goodness is lost.
- Ginger. Apart from its numerous medicinal properties, ginger is a known anti-inflammatory substance, so it can be very good for Rheumatoid Arthritis.

- Grains. C-reactive protein is a known marker for inflammation. Whole grains such as brown rice, oatmeal, and cereals help to lower the content of this C-reactive protein in the blood, thus preventing its onset and flare-ups.

- Grapes. There is no doubt that fruits are very nutritious. Grapes are high in antioxidants that can bring a reduction in the development of various inflammatory symptoms. It contains resveratrol which is found on the skin of grapes; and it is believed to help patients by preventing RA cells from forming. Finally, it contains proanthocyanidin which effectively reduces inflammation relate to Rheumatoid Arthritis.

- Green Tea. It is rich in polyphenols and antioxidants; it is have reliable anti-inflammatory properties that can relieve patients of debilitating symptoms and also slow down the rate of cartilage destruction. Apart from that it also contains epigallocatechin-3-gallate (EGCG) to block the attack of molecules that causes destruction in the joints.
- Nuts. Rich in calcium, zinc, magnesium, protein, vitamin E and alpha linolenic acid (ALA), nuts like pistachios, walnuts, almonds and pine nuts are very good for an immune system boost.

Recommended consumption is about 1.5 oz daily

- Oils. Extra virgin oil is not only good for the heart, but it has a special component called oleocanthal, that behaves very much like your NSAIDs (non steroidal anti-inflammatory drugs). Plant-based and nut oils such as safflower oil, avocado oil, and walnut oil are offer an array of benefits. They are a rich source of omega-3 fatty acids.

Recommended consumption is about 2 to 3 tbsp daily
- Oranges. Rich in vitamin C, oranges as well as other citrus fruits like limes and grapefruits helps prevent the onset of Rheumatoid Arthritis.

- Parsley. Popular as a garnish, it contains luteolin that has the ability to block the action of inflammatory proteins. It is, therefore, able to deal with the symptoms related to Rheumatoid Arthritis.

- Pineapple. The most people are fond of it, but the stem of the pineapple contains bromelain. This substance has very impressive anti-inflammatory properties, and will serve beneficial against the symptoms of RA.

- Pomegranates. Rich in anthocyanin which is a flavonoid that is an effective in combating inflammation. It is also rich in antioxidants which can give protection to the attack of free radiacals.

- Soy beans. Another great source of omega-3 fatty acids, soy beans can take the place of fish for those who are not too fond of them. The best sources of soy are edamame and tofu. It is high in protein and fiber, but low in fat, so it is very good for you.

- Spinach. Leafy vegetables are very nutritious. Spinach is rich in antioxidants that will not only combat the disease, but also help provide relief against the symptoms related to inflammation. It is also rich in kaempferol which reduces inflammation related to RA and osteoarthritis.

Your Rheumatoid Anti-Inflammatory Diet Plan

So what exactly is the best diet for RA sufferers? The main issue with Rheumatoid Arthritis is inflammation. Studies show that maintaining a plant-based diet results in the decrease of the accumulation of a certain protein that causes the symptoms of RA. Maintaining a predominantly vegan diet has been found to be truly beneficial to sufferers.

The main problem is inflammation so the main diet is supposed to be, anti-inflammatory. It should be consist of food that has the capacity to prevent, reduce, and/or alleviate the onset and symptoms of inflammation.

Your Anti-Inflammatory Diet plan resolves around food such as fish, vegetables, and oils. Your perfect diet against Rheumatoid Arthritis is either of the two:

Mediterranean Diet

Researches show that the best diet for Rheumatoid Arthritis is the Mediterranean Diet. This diet is rich in nutrients with the specific action of reducing the onset of inflammation in the body, so maintaining it will help you deal not only with the symptoms, but also with the condition.
Patients not only see a decrease in inflammatory episodes, but they personally experience increased physical function within affected joints.

Vegetarian Diet

Going vegetarian is not only a healthy choice, but with a diet low in arachidonic acid, patients suffering from Rheumatoid Arthritis observed that their inflammatory episodes have been more bearable or have generally lessened due to the diet.

Chapter 6: One Week Diet Plan for Patients with Rheumatoid Arthritis

In Chapter 5, the book looked into specific foods that patients with Rheumatoid Arthritis need to avoid and have more of. In the general sense, your winning diet against RA is one that lowers your AGE – advanced glycation end product. AGE is a toxin that is found very high in pasteurized, fried, processed, heated, and grilled food. When your diet is high in AGE, your body will release a lot of cytokines in an effort to attack them. This defensive mechanism only results in unnecessary increased inflammatory activity that will only bring damage to the body.

The Mediterranean Diet

While there is not specific diet that addresses the problem perfectly, the features of a Mediterranean Diet support the necessity that sufferers need in order to leave comfortably with their condition.

Day 1

Breakfast: Cinnamon and Pear Oatmeal with Egg

¼ cup pears, chopped
½ tsp cinnamon
1 egg
¼ cup oats
1 tbsp sugar
¼ cup vanilla yogurt
salt, to taste

1. In a bowl, combine the egg and milk. Beat them together and add the pears oats, sugar, cinnamon, and salt.

2. Boil the egg mixture until the liquid is fully absorbed.

3. Top it with yogurt and chopped pears, to serve.

Lunch: Chicken with Spinach and Artichoke Pasta

14 oz artichoke hearts, drained and chopped
1 lb chicken breast fillet, skinned and cubed
½ cup feta cheese, crumbled
2 cloves garlic, crushed
3 tbsp lemon juice
2 lemons, wedged (for garnish)
1 ½ tbsp olive oil
1 cup onion, chopped
2 tsp dried oregano
3 tbsp parsley, chopped
16 oz linguini pasta
1 ½ cup spinach, coarsely chopped
1 tomato, chopped
salt and pepper, to taste

1. In a pot, boil pasta according to package instructions.

2. In a skillet, heat oil ad sauté garlic and onion until translucent, then add the chicken and cook thoroughly.

3. Add the tomatoes, artichoke hearts, spinach, feta cheese, oregano, lemon juice, and parsley. Add the cooked pasta and mix everything well. Season with salt and pepper.

4. Serve with a garnish of lemon wedges.

Dinner: Chickpea, Edamame and Kidney Bean Salad

1 tsp capers, drained
15.5 oz chickpeas, drained
15 oz edamame
15 oz kidney beans, drained
1 lemon, zested and juiced

3 tbsp extra virgin olive il
½ cup onion, chopped
½ cup parsley, chopped
1 tomato, chopped
 salt, to taste

1. In a bowl, combine the beans, lemon zest and juice, capers, parsley, tomatoes, olive oil, and salt.

2. Mix well and cover to refrigerate for about 2 hours.

3. Toss well before serving.

Dessert: Mixed Berries, Banana and Avocado Smoothie

2 ripe avocadoes, seeded and quartered
1 banana, frozen and quartered
2 cups mixed berries, frozen
ice water, as needed
maple syrup and agave, to taste

1. In a blender, combine frozen berries, bananas, and avocados with ¼ cup ice water. Let things run until smooth.

2. Add maple syrup or agave to taste. Discard berry seeds before serving.

Day 2

Breakfast: Quinoa and Avocado Cheese Breakfast Medley

½ avocado, peeled, seeded and diced
1 tsp basil
¼ cup feta cheese, crumbled
¼ cup Parmesan cheese
8 eggs
1 ½ cups non-fat milk
olive oil spray
½ tsp oregano
½ cup spinach, chopped
½ tsp thyme
¼ cup sundried tomatoes
½ cup uncooked quinoa
salt, to taste

1. Preheat oven to 350°F

2. In a bowl, combine milk, eggs, avocado, dun dried tomatoes, feta cheese thyme, spinach, quinoa, basil, oregano, and salt. Pour this mixture into a quiche dish and cover it with foil.

3. Pop it into the oven and let it bake for about 45 minutes to an hour.

4. Take the dish out, sprinkle Parmesan cheese on top and then return it to the oven and let it bake for 10-15 minutes.

Lunch: Mediterranean Flounder Fish with Tomatoes

6, 6 basil leaves, chopped and torn
¼ cup capers
3 tbsp Parmesan cheese, grated
1 lb flounder fish, fillet

2 cloves garlic, chopped
1 tsp lemon juice
1 pinch Italian seasoning
24 kalamata olives, pitted and chopped
2 tbsp extra virgin olive oil
½ onion, chopped
5 plum tomatoes
¼ cup white wine

1. Preheat oven to 425°F.

2. In a saucepan, let water boil and drop the tomatoes in, then collect them again and leave them in an ice water bath, so you can easily tear off the skin. Dice the tomatoes. Set it aside.

3. In a skillet, heat oil and sauté the onions until tender. Add the diced tomatoes, Italian seasoning, and garlic. Cook until the tomatoes are tender.

4. Add the wine, olives, lemon juice, capers, ½ of the basil and reduce the heat. Add the Parmesan cheese and continue cooking until the sauce becomes thick.

5. In a baking dish, lay the flounder fish, and pour the sauce over it. Sprinkle the remaining basil leaves on top. Pop the dish into the oven and let the fish bake until it is cooked through.

Dinner: Zesty Sweet Potatoes and Zucchini Casserole

½ lemon, juiced
½ cup olive oil
4 onions, thinly sliced
2 tbsp parsley, chopped
2 lbs sweet potatoes, peeled and sliced
6 tomatoes, crushed
1tsp turmeric, ground
4 zucchini, sliced

salt and pepper, to taste

1. Preheat oven to 400°F.

2. In a baking dish, spread the zucchini, potatoes and
    onions. Spread evenly and cover everything with the
    crushed tomatoes, then top it with parsley and olive oil.
    Season it with salt and pepper then pops the dish into
    the oven.

3. Bake for about an hour. Make sure to stir occasionally.

Dessert: Avocado Cinnamon Cookies

1 ripe avocado, peeled and seeded
½ tsp cinnamon, ground
½ tsp baking powder
½ tsp baking soda
4 oz butter, unsalted
1 egg
1 cup whole wheat flour
1tsp nutmeg
1 ½ cup old fashioned oats
1 ¼ cup raisins
¼ cup sugar
½ cup dark brown sugar

1. Preheat oven to 325°F.

2. On a baking dish, arrange the oats and let them toast in
    the oven, until they are golden. Set it aside to cool.
3. Line the baking dish with aluminum foil. In a bowl, sift
    the baking soda and baking powder. Set it aside.

4. In an electric mixer, blend the butter until it is creamed.
    Add both white and brown sugar, by increments. Add
    egg to the mixture and continue to blend it. Add the
    avocado and blend it well with the oats. Finally, add the
    raisins, nutmeg, and cinnamon.

5. Shape cookies on the lined baking dish. Pop them into the oven until they are browned. Then let them cool before serving.

Day 3

Breakfast: Cheesy Eggs with Green Peppercorns

1 tsp dried basil
¼ cup dry breadcrumbs, divided
½ Swiss chard
½ cup goat cheese, crumbled
4 eggs
3 tbsp extra virgin olive oil
1 tsp dried oregano
1 ½ tsp green peppercorns, coarsely crushed
2 shallots, finely chopped
2 plum tomatoes, chopped
1 tbsp water
salt, to taste

1. Take the Swiss chard. Remove the center rib and stems. Cut them in half and them crosswise. Set aside.

2. Preheat oven to 400°F.

3. Grease custard cups or ramekins and sprinkle the bottom with breadcrumbs.

4. In a skillet, heat oil and sauté the shallots, peppercorns and salt until the vegetables are tender.

5. Add the Swiss chard and water. Continue cooking until the liquid evaporates. Spoon about a ¼ cup of the Swiss chard mixture into the greased ramekins or cups then top it with tomatoes. Finally, gently place one egg on

top, making sure not to break the yolk. Sprinkle with goat cheese and season with salt.

6. Pop the dish into the oven and let it bake for about 16 to 18 minutes. Let it stand before serving.

Lunch: Avocado Basket with Tuna in Balsamic Vinegar

2 ripe avocados, halved and pitted
1 dash balsamic vinegar
1 red bell pepper, chopped
4 onions, thinly sliced
1 tbsp mayonnaise
12 oz white tuna in water, drained
salt and pepper, to taste

1. In a bowl, combine tuna, onions, mayonnaise, red bell pepper, tuna, and balsamic vinegar. Mix well and season it with salt and pepper.

2. Pack the avocado halves with the tuna mixture and garnish it with onions and black pepper to serve.

Dinner: Sweet Radish and Walnut Salad

1 tsp honey
2 tsp lemon juice
20 fresh mint leaves
3 tbsp extra virgin olive oil
1 lb radishes, trimmed and sliced
¾ tsp salt
1 ½ cups walnut, halved

1. In a skillet, toast walnuts until fragrant. Cool and chop.

2. In a small bowl, combine the lemon juice, oil, honey and salt. Mix well.

3. In a large bowl, toss the radishes with the prepared dressing; Make sure to coat everything evenly.

4. Slice the mint leaves and toss them into a bowl with the walnuts. Finally, fold the mint and walnuts into the prepared salad.

Dessert: Fruit and Nut Biscotti

½ cup avocado, mashed
2 tbsp baking soda
1 ½ cups cranberries
3 eggs
3 cups all-purpose flour
2 tbsp lemon juice
1 tbsp low-fat milk
1/3 fresh cup orange juice
3 tsp grated orange peel
½ cup pistachios, unshelled
1 tsp salt
¾ cup sugar
2 tsp vanilla extract

1. Preheat oven to 325°F. Line a baking sheet with parchment paper.

2. In a pan, combine orange juice and cranberries and let it boil. Add the orange peel and then slowly fold the baking soda, flour and salt with the mixture. Set it aside.

3. In a bowl, combine the avocado, sugar, and lemon juice. Add the eggs, one at a time, and beat it well until smooth. Add the vanilla extract and blend it well until smooth.

4. Add the orange-cranberry mixture prepared earlier. Combine the pistachio nuts and mix everything well together.

5. Knead the dough and form them into logs that are about ½ inch thick and 4 inches wide. Coat the top of the logs with milk. Lay them on the baking sheet and pop them into the oven. Let it bake for about 35 minutes.

6. Let it cool and slice them into ½ thick pieces then bring them back to the oven to toast for about 15 minutes (on each side). Let it cool before serving.

Day 4

Breakfast: Zucchini Frittata with Mozza Balls

2 ½ oz mozzarella balls
8 eggs
1 tbsp olive oil
½ tsp red pepper, crushed
½ cup cherry tomatoes, halved
½ cup walnuts, coarsely chopped
1 zucchini, thinly sliced
salt, to taste

1. Preheat broiler.

2. In a bowl, combine eggs, crushed red peppers, and salt together.

3. In a skillet, heat oil and lay the zucchini slices evenly. Cook them until they soften, then top it with cherry tomatoes. Cook for about 3-5 minutes.

4. Add the egg mixture then top it with walnuts and mozzarella balls. Let it broil for 3 minutes before serving.

Lunch: Crispy Chickpea Falafel

¼ tsp baking soda
15 oz chickpea, rinsed and drained
¼ tsp coriander, ground
2 tsp cumin, ground
1 egg, beaten
1 tbsp all-purpose flour
4 cloves garlic, minced
2 tsp olive oil
¼ cup onion, chopped
½ cup parsley, chopped
salt, to taste

1. Preheat oven to 400°F.

2. Wrap onions in a cheese cloth and squeeze it to dehydrate. Set it aside.

3. In a food processor, combine the chickpeas, parsley, cumin, baking soda, garlic, coriander, and salt. Let it run until coarsely pureed.

4. In a bowl, combine the chickpea puree with the dehydrated onions and shape this mixture into large patties

5. In an oven-safe skillet, heat oil and cook the patties until they are golden brown. Pop the skillet into the oven and let it bake for about 10 minutes.

6. Serve with whole wheat pita bread.

Dinner: Herb Lentil Soup

2 bay leaves
1 pinch basil
1 carrot, chopped
1 tbsp garlic, minced

8 oz brown lentil
¼ cup, 1 tsp olive oil
1 onion, minced
1 pinch oregano
1 pinch rosemary
1 pinch thyme
1 tsp red wine vinegar
1 tbsp tomato paste
1 quart water
salt and pepper, to taste

1. In a saucepan, boil the lentils until tender, making sure that the water is about an inch high. Drain water and set aside.

2. In the same saucepan, heat oil and sauté garlic and onions until tender. Add the carrots and stir fry until softened, then add the lentils. Add the water, rosemary, oregano, and bay leaves. Let things simmer for about 10 minutes.

3. Add tomato paste and season everything with salt and pepper. Let it simmer until the lentils have softened, making sure to stir from time to time. You may add more water if the lentils go dry.

4. Drizzle with 1 tsp olive oil and red wine vinegar before serving.

Dessert: Sweet Pear and Nut Medley Basket

3 tsp almond, chopped
3 tbsp cashews, chopped
2 tbsp lemon juice
8 pears, peeled
½ cup raisins
5 tbsp honey
6 tbsp walnuts, chopped
½ cup water

1. Preheat oven to 350°F.

2. Cut the pears in half, taking out the core.

3. In a small bowl, combine the walnuts, raisins, sugar, and lemon juice. Mix everything well together. Scoop a spoonful of this mixture into the pear halves. You may or may not drizzle some honey on top.

4. Pop the pears into the oven and let it bake with foil on top, for about 1 hour and 15 minutes.

Day 5

Breakfast: Asparagus and Avocado Whole Wheat Sandwich

12 asparagus spears
1 avocado, peeled and mashed
1 egg, boiled and sliced
olive oil
4 slices whole wheat bread, toasted
Dijon mustard, to taste
salt and pepper, to taste

1. Spread mustard on two slices of bread. Spread mashed avocado on the other two slices.

2. Assemble the sandwich by laying asparagus and egg slices on the avocado side. Sprinkle the top with salt and pepper, and then drizzle it with olive oil. Cover the sandwich.

Lunch: Quinoa and Kalamata Chicken Salad

1 green bell pepper, diced
½ cup feta cheese, crumbled

2 ½ chicken breast fillet, cubed
½ cup chives, chopped
2 cubes chicken bouillon
1 clove garlic, crushed
2/3 cup lemon juice
1 cup kalamata olives, chopped
¼ cup olive oil
1 onion, diced
½ cup parsley, chopped
1 cup quinoa, uncooked
1 tbsp balsamic vinegar
2 cups water
salt, to taste

1. In a saucepan, boil the bouillon cubes and the garlic. Add the quinoa and let it simmer until all the water has been absorbed. Discard the garlic. Transfer the quinoa to a bowl.

2. Add the chicken, bell pepper, onion, feta cheese, olives, chives, parsley, and salt into the boiled quinoa. Mix evenly and drizzle it with balsamic vinegar, olive oil, and lemon juice.

3. Serve warm or cold.

Dinner: Chicken and Sausage with Rosemary

1 red bell pepper, thinly sliced
8 chicken breast fillets, halved
1 ½ tbsp cornstarch
5 cloves garlic, minced
1 onion, thinly sliced
1 tsp oregano
½ cup parsley, chopped
2 tsp rosemary
8 oz turkey Italian sausages
¼ cup dry vermouth
2 tbsp cold water
salt and pepper, to taste

1. In a slow cooker, combine the bell pepper, onion, garlic, oregano, and rosemary. Mix well and add the crumbled sausages. Finally, add the chicken on top of the sausages and season everything with pepper. Finally add the vermouth and cover it cooker. Leave everything until chicken is tender.

2. Transfer the chicken to a warm dish and set it aside. Leave the sauce in the cooker.

3. In a small bowl, combine cold water and cornstarch. Add it to the sauce in the cooker and let it cook until it thickens. Season with salt.

4. Cover the chicken with the sauce and serve.

Dessert: Zesty Olive Cake

1 tsp baking powder
1 tsp baking soda
2 tsp cardamom, ground
2 tsp cinnamon, ground
1 tsp cloves, ground
1 cup currants
3 eggs
2 tbsp fennel seeds
2 cups whole wheat flour
1 cup crystallized ginger, diced.
½ cup extra virgin olive oil
2 cups black olives, pitted and chopped
1 orange, juiced and zested
3 tbsp pomegranate molasses
1 cup plain Greek yogurt

1. Preheat oven to 350ºF. Grease cake pan and line with parchment paper.

2. In a bowl, combine baking soda, baking powder, flour, cinnamon, cardamom, and cloves. Blend everything with a whisk and set it aside.

3. In another bowl, combine the eggs, yogurt, olive oil, 2 tbsp pomegranate molasses. Mix everything well and add the dry ingredients.

4. Fold in the orange zest, olives, currants, fennel seeds, and ginger. Mix everything well until smooth.

5. Spoon batter into the greased pan and pop it into the oven. Let it bake for about 35 to 40 minutes or until a toothpick comes out cleanly.

6. In a saucepan, combine orange juice, the remaining molasses and let it simmer. Add sugar and whisk it well until the mixture glazes. Pour the glaze over the cake before serving.

Day 6

Breakfast: Kale Egg White Frittata with Goat Cheese

1 ½ oz goat cheese, crumbled
6 eggs
4 egg whites
2 ½ cups kale, coarsely torn
2 tsp olive oil
1 onion, sliced
½ cup sun-dried tomatoes, sliced
salt and pepper, to taste

1. Preheat broiler.

2. In an oven-proof skillet, stir fry onions and kale, until the onions are tender.

3. In a bowl, combine the egg whites, eggs, salt, and pepper. Pout this mixture over the kale and onions. Cook everything in medium heat.

4. Once the mixture sets, run a spatula around the edge of the skillet while cooking and make sure to egg remains moist and glossy.

5. Top this with goat cheese and dried tomatoes. Let it broil until the eggs are set.

Lunch: Feta Cheese and Mushroom Bake

½ cup feta cheese, crumbled
2 tbsp Parmesan cheese, grated
4 mushrooms, sliced
3 tbsp olive oil
6 whole wheat pita bread
1 bunch spinach, chopped
6 oz sun-dried tomato pesto
2 plum tomatoes, chopped
pepper, to taste

1. Preheat oven to 350°F.

2. Spread tomato pesto on one side of each pita bread and lay them on a baking sheet.

3. On top of each, arrange spinach, tomatoes, mushrooms, feta cheese and Parmesan cheese. Drizzle it with olive oil. Add a dash of pepper on top.

4. Pop the dish into the oven and bake until the pita bread are crisp.

Dinner: Shrimp and Tomato Penne Pasta

1 cup Parmesan cheese, grated
2 tbsp garlic, chopped

2 tbsp olive oil
½ cup onion, chopped
16 oz penne pasta
1 ½ lbs shrimp, peeled and deveined
14.5 oz tomatoes, diced
¼ cup white wine

1. In a large pot, boil pasta according to package instructions.

2. In a skillet, heat oil and sauté onion and garlic until tender.

3. Add the tomatoes and wine and cook everything for about 10 minutes. Make sure to stir from time to time. Add the shrimps and cook until opaque.

4. Add everything to the cooked pasta. Add Parmesan cheese before serving.

Dessert: Mixed Berry Bulgur with Ginger Zest

¼ cup blackberries
¼ cup blueberries
¼ cup strawberries
¼ cup bulgur
3 tbsp coconut milk
1 tbsp crystallized ginger
2 tbsp honey
2/3 low-fat Greek yogurt

1. In a bowl, combine the yogurt, bulgur, coconut milk money and ginger together. Mix well and divide it into two jars.

2. Top it with chopped berries, cover the lid and let it chill overnight, in the freezer. You may chill it up to three days.

3. Stir loosely before serving.

Day 7

Breakfast: Sweet Pea and Edamame Wrap

1 cup edamame, cooked
2 eggs
2 cloves garlic, minced
2 tbsp lemon juice
2 ½ tbsp mint, chopped
2 tbsp, 2 tsp extra virgin olive oil
1 cup sweet peas, cooked
2 tbsp tahini
2 whole wheat tortillas

1. In a food processor, combine edamame, sweet peas, 1 tbsp olive oil, tahini, lemon juice, mint and garlic. Blend everything until smooth. Spread it evenly on one side of the tortillas.

2. In a skillet, heat remaining oil and fry the eggs. Place the eggs on top of the arranged tortillas. Feel free to garnish the top with any remaining peas, edamame, or mint.

Lunch: Caramelized Italian Sausage Pasta

1 green bell pepper, sliced
1 red bell pepper, sliced
1 clove garlic, minced
1 onion, sliced
1 pinch oregano
16 oz bow tie pasta
1lb mild Italian sausage links
14.5 oz Italian-style tomatoes, diced
1/3 cup water
1 tbsp Marsala wine
pepper, to taste

1. In a large pot, cook pasta according to package instructions.

2. In a skillet, boil the sausages in 1/3 cup water. Drain and slice.

3. In the same skillet, heat oil and return the boiled sausages. Add the onions, garlic, peppers, and Marsala wine. Add the diced tomatoes, oregano, and black pepper. Serve it over the pasta.

Dinner: Spinach and Bean Soup

16 oz white kidney beans, rinsed and drained
1 celery, chopped
14 oz chicken broth
2 cloves garlic, minced
2 tbsp lemon juice
1 ½ onion, chopped
1 bunch spinach, thinly sliced
¼ tsp thyme
1 tbsp vegetable oil
2 cups water
pepper, to taste

1. In a saucepan, heat oil and sauté celery and onion until tender. Add garlic.

2. Add the beans, thyme, chicken broth, pepper, and 2 cups water. Bring everything to a boil and then let it simmer for about 15 minutes. Gather about 2 cups of this mixture and set it aside.

3. In a blender, let the remaining mixture of the soup run until it is smooth, and then bring it back to the pot. Return the reserved bean mixture.

4. Let everything boil, making sure to stir it from time to time. Add spinach and cook it until it is wilted. Finally add lemon juice.

5. Remove from heat and top it with Parmesan cheese to serve.

Dessert: Date and Almond Smoothie

1 ½ banana
2 tbsp almond butter
½ cup medjool dates, pitted
1 ½ tbsp honey
1 cup ice cubes
2 cups almond milk, unsweetened

1. In a bowl, combine the dates and milk together. Cover it and let it chill, overnight, in the freezer.

2. In a blender, combine dates, milk, almond butter, and honey. Blend well until smooth. Add ice and continue running it in the blender until your reach the right consistency.

Why Should You Go Mediterranean?

The Mediterranean Diet has Greek and Italian origins. While this book focuses on the capacity of this diet to improve the lives of people suffering from Rheumatoid Arthririts, it is also believed that the healthy features of this diet go beyond joint, bone, and cartilage health.

Chapter 7: Living with Rheumatoid Arthritis

There is no cure for Rheumatoid Arthritis, but it does not mean that your situation is hopeless. There are ways for you to cope with the condition, so that you can live comfortably. The role of diet and supplementation has been discussed in the previous chapters. In this Chapter, you will learn more valuable tips that will help you through your journey.

Therapies and Activities that Alleviate Symptoms

The symptoms of Rheumatoid Arthritis are most problematic when the joints are being used. Unfortunately, being immobile is not an option, if you want to continue living your life. The injury that the symptoms of RA bring to the body, have the capacity to change people's lives. The following therapies and activities can help make things normal:

1. Exercise. Exercise is very good for patients with RA, but since mobility is fairly minimal, it is best that you choose activities that will subject the least trauma to the patient. Rheumatoid Arthritis can be very devastating, but with regular exercise, you can maintain mobility within the joints and strengthen the muscles around the area. Yoga, biking, walking, swimming, and tai chi is great for developing strength and flexibility. Apart from its physical benefits, regular exercise can help deal with the emotional damage this problem brings.

2. Acupuncture. Very popular in the East, acupuncture involves the stimulation of certain points on the body with the use of tiny needles. The needles are inserted into the skin and left there for a few minutes to about an hour, to attract specific energies to the body. Proper acupuncture helps in the release of certain "feel good" hormones that definitely help in the management of the symptoms of Rheumatoid Arthritis.

3. Physical therapy. If there is extreme loss of mobility due to RA, you can help make things better with physical therapy. A physical therapist uses various methods to help a patient. Some of the modalities include transcutaneous electrical stimulation, ice, heat, range-of-motion exercises, and strengthening exercises. This is a short-term address, and those who undergo this will have to see the PT, several times in a week. Most people go for PT so that they can improve their mobility and carryout exercises on their own.

4. Occupational therapy. When you employ the services of an occupational therapist, they will help you identify your problems so that you can work around it. If you need help with the use of your hands and wrists, to be able to continue working, they will help transform your work area to support your specific need.

5. Massage. RA involves painful and tender joints—so to bring some ease to the tensed muscles and joint areas; massage of varying pressures can be quite beneficial.

6. Mind-body therapy. Mind over matter suggests that there are things in this world that can be achieved through various mind-body techniques. Strategies within this discipline include biofeedback, mindful meditation, breathing exercises, and guided relaxation. Such methods help patients cope not only with the pain and discomfort; and it helps improve flexibility and strength.

7. Temperature and pressure. The oldest remedy for Rheumatoid Arthritis has to do with temperature. Enjoying a hot shower or bath is not just relaxing, but it is able to soothe ailing joints to be able to achieve some relief. Cold or warm compress is also useful. One can do alternating applications of both cold and warm packs on the area in question, to get some relief from pain and discomfort.

8. Rest. Believe it or not, rest in its simplicity is a very valuable RA remedy. The joints are will only ache more when they are not given ample rest. So if you want your condition to improve, you can give yourself some rest.

Support Group and Therapy

When the effects of RA have gone beyond the superficial problem, the patient will require emotional support. Individually, one can make a decision to go into counseling to undergo psychotherapy. The effects of Rheumatoid Arthritis, especially with patients that have plummeted to depression, can be quite catastrophic. This makes the condition more than a physical disability, because those who aren't able to cope with the effects developmental problems, as well.

Cognitive behavioral therapy is a psychotherapy that helps sufferers deal with the emotional turmoil involved in the condition. Patients can attend counseling sessions, either as an individual or with a group, in order to gain liberation from RA.

Conclusion

Rheumatoid Arthritis is not going to be a walk in the park, but when treatment is consistent and approach is more holistic, a patient can enjoy a very comfortable life. It can be debilitating, but the condition is fairly manageable when it is detected earlier in its development.

Prevention of Rheumatoid Arthritis

There are so many risk factors that predispose a person to developing Rheumatoid Arthritis, but mostly RA is an autoimmune disease and when there is a malfunction in the body system, it can wreak havoc.

Suffice it to say, it is not going to be easy pin point that will develop RA, but this book more or less focused on the most important thing: to change the way you live.

- Control your diet in such a way, so that your body is not prone to inflammation. Equip yourself with the dietary knowledge that supports your fight against RA, by strictly avoiding the food that cause inflammation and having more the substances that are good for you. The simple cutting of sugar from your diet is already beneficial. Switch to a Mediterranean-type diet so you can take advantage of its great benefits.

- Avoid stress. The function of the immune system is heavily compromised when you are subjected to a lot of stress. Stress causes the release of cytokines that causes inflammation. Inasmuch as you can, try to avoid stressful activities and situations. Engage in distressing activities such as meditation and yoga, to be able to lessen the stress in your life and avoid the onset of Rheumatoid Arthritis.

- Quit smoking. Cigarette smoking is such an awful habit. And if you a smoker, you are increasing your risk of developing RA. The chemicals contained in a stick of cigarette can do so much damage to your body. Get rid of your cigarettes and by doing so you do not only save yourself from the debilitating symptoms of RA, you also give yourself a healthier chance at life.

- Lose weight. If you are overweight or obese, it is time to cut down. An anti-inflammatory diet offers a good weight loss benefit; but it is best when you include exercise in your weight loss regime. There is a better chance of suffering worn out joints when you are overweight, so try to cut down.

Basically, you have to make a commitment to live a life that supports your needs. Rheumatoid Arthritis remains without a cure but to prevent its onset or prevent flare-ups from controlling your life, you need to take control of the whole situation.

Traditional treatments and over-the-counter medications have been the world's go-to solution, but for a chronic illness such as RA, you cannot carelessly depend on medicines. The harmful side-effects that are part and parcel of the whole ordeal should be enough to convince you to stay away and take a more natural direction. This book takes you through the whole journey, so that you can deal with Rheumatoid Arthritis without having to rely with harmful chemicals.

Natural is safe. Going natural helps you deal with the problem, holistically. Hopefully this book changes your life so that you can gain control of your condition, and not the other way around.